This book belongs to

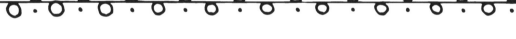

D1609361

Contents

PAGE

Birth INFORMATION

Name			
Date		Weight	
Time		Length	
Place of birth		Head circumference	
Doctor			
Nurse			

Blood group	
Parents name	
Home address	
Phone No	
Email address	

Notes

Medical CONTACT INFORMATION

PRIMARY CARE PHYSICIAN

Name	
Address	
Phone No	

PEDIATRICIAN

Name	
Address	
Phone No	

DENTIST

Name	
Address	
Phone No	

PHARMACIST

Name	
Address	
Phone No	

Medical CONTACT INFORMATION

SPECIALIST:

Name	
Address	
Phone No	

SPECIALIST:

Name	
Address	
Phone No	

SPECIALIST:

Name	
Address	
Phone No	

SPECIALIST:

Name	
Address	
Phone No	

Growth CHART

Date	Age	Weight	Height	Note

Growth CHART

Date	Age	Weight	Height	Note

Growth CHART

Date	Age	Weight	Height	Note

Baby MILESTONES

Milestones	Date	Age	Notes
Smile			
Held head up			

Baby MILESTONES

Milestones	Date	Age	Notes

$\mathcal{B}aby$ MILESTONES

Milestones	Date	Age	Notes

Tooth BABY CHART

Write in the date for each new tooth

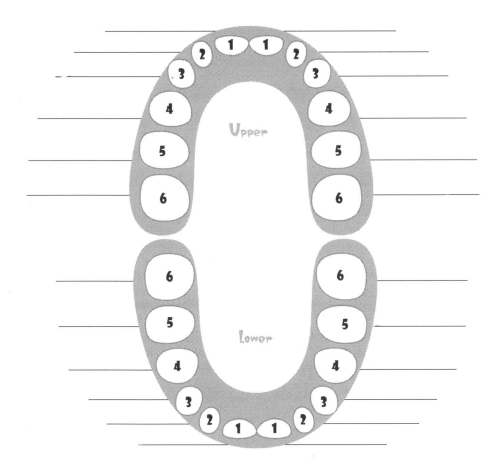

Tooth	Upper	Lower
1. central Incisor	8-12 months	6-10 months
2. lateral incisor	9-13 months	10-16 months
3. cuspid	16-22 months	17-23 months
4. first molar	13-19 months	14-18 months
5. second molar	25-33 months	23-31 months
6. first permanent molar	6-7 years	6-7 years

Permanent TEETH

Write in the date for each new tooth

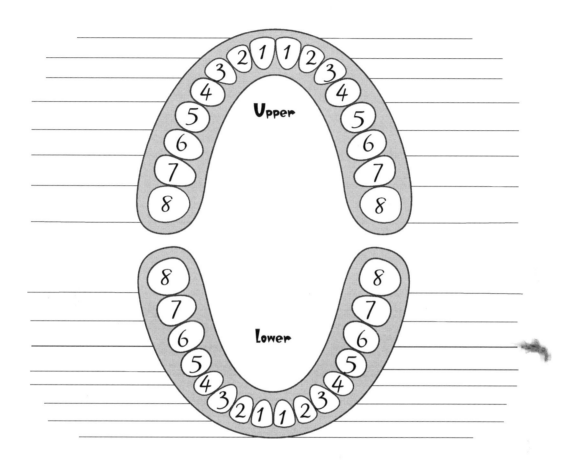

Tooth	Upper	Lower
1. Central Incisor	7–8 yrs	7–8 yrs
2. Lateral Incisor	8–9 yrs	8–9 yrs
3. Canine (Cuspid, Eye Tooth)	11–12 yrs	11–12 yrs
4. First Premolar	10–11 yrs	10–11 yrs
5. Second Premolar	10–12 yrs	10–12 yrs
6. First Molar (6-yr molar)	6–7 yrs	6–7 yrs
7. Second Molar (12-yr Molar)	12–13 yrs	12–13 yrs
8. Third Molar (Wisdom Tooth)	17–21 yrs	17–21 yrs

Vaccination RECORDS

Vaccine	Dates			

Vaccination RECORDS

Vaccine	Dates			

Vaccination RECORDS

Vaccine	Dates			

Vaccination RECORDS

Vaccine	*Dates*			

Family HISTORY

Do this diseases run in your family?

MEDICAL CONDITION	YES	HOW MANY PEOPLE
Diabetes	○	
High blood Pressure	○	
Heart disease	○	
Stroke	○	
High cholesterol	○	
Alzheimer's Disease	○	
Mental Illness	○	
Kidney Problems	○	
Liver Disease	○	
Lung Disease	○	
Thyroid Disease	○	
Arthritis	○	
GastroIntestinal Disease	○	
Depression	○	
Auto immune disease	○	
Birth defects	○	
Infertility	○	
endometriosis	○	
Blood Disease	○	
Epilepsy	○	
Allergies	○	
Tumors/Cancer	○	
Congenital Heart Disorder	○	

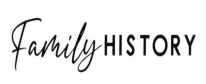

Family HISTORY

FAMILY MEMBERS	ILLNESS	DESCRIBE

Family HISTORY

FAMILY MEMBERS	ILLNESS	DESCRIBE

$\mathscr{Symptom}$ **TRACKER**

Date	Time	Symptom	Notes

Symptom TRACKER

Date	Time	Symptom	Notes

Symptom TRACKER

Date	Time	Symptom	Notes

Symptom TRACKER

Date	Time	Symptom	Notes

Symptom TRACKER

Date	Time	Symptom	Notes

Symptom TRACKER

Date	Time	Symptom	Notes

Symptom TRACKER

Date	Time	Symptom	Notes

Symptom TRACKER

Date	Time	Symptom	Notes

Symptom TRACKER

Date	Time	Symptom	Notes

Symptom TRACKER

Date	Time	Symptom	Notes

Symptom TRACKER

Date	Time	Symptom	Notes

Symptom TRACKER

Date	Time	Symptom	Notes

Symptom TRACKER

Date	Time	Symptom	Notes

Symptom TRACKER

Date	Time	Symptom	Notes

Symptom TRACKER

Date	Time	Symptom	Notes

Symptom TRACKER

Date	Time	Symptom	Notes

Symptom TRACKER

Date	Time	Symptom	Notes

Symptom TRACKER

Date	Time	Symptom	Notes

Symptom TRACKER

Date	Time	Symptom	Notes

Symptom TRACKER

Date	Time	Symptom	Notes

Symptom TRACKER

Date	Time	Symptom	Notes

Symptom TRACKER

Date	Time	Symptom	Notes

Symptom TRACKER

Date	Time	Symptom	Notes

Symptom TRACKER

Date	Time	Symptom	Notes

Symptom TRACKER

Date	Time	Symptom	Notes

Symptom TRACKER

Date	Time	Symptom	Notes

Symptom TRACKER

Date	Time	Symptom	Notes

Symptom TRACKER

Date	Time	Symptom	Notes

Symptom TRACKER

Date	Time	Symptom	Notes

Symptom TRACKER

Date	Time	Symptom	Notes

Doctor VISIT LOG

Date		Time	
Doctor		Contact	
Location			

REASON FOR VISIT

QUESTIONS/NOTES

DIAGNOSIS/FEEDBACK

PRESCRIPTION/INSTRUCTION

Temperature		Heart rate	
Weight		Blood pressure	

NOTES:---

Doctor VISIT LOG

Date		Time	
Doctor		Contact	
Location			

REASON FOR VISIT

QUESTIONS/NOTES

DIAGNOSIS/FEEDBACK

PRESCRIPTION/INSTRUCTION

Temperature		Heart rate	
Weight		Blood pressure	

NOTES:------------------------------------

Doctor VISIT LOG

Date		Time	
Doctor		Contact	
Location			

REASON FOR VISIT

QUESTIONS/NOTES

DIAGNOSIS/FEEDBACK

PRESCRIPTION/INSTRUCTION

Temperature		Heart rate	
Weight		Blood pressure	

NOTES: --

Doctor VISIT LOG

Date		Time	
Doctor		Contact	
Location			

REASON FOR VISIT

- -
- -
- -
- -
- -

QUESTIONS/NOTES

- -
- -
- -
- -
- -

DIAGNOSIS/FEEDBACK

- -
- -
- -
- -
- -

PRESCRIPTION/INSTRUCTION

- -
- -
- -
- -
- -

Temperature		Heart rate	
Weight		Blood pressure	

NOTES: -
- -
- -
- -

Doctor VISIT LOG

Date		Time	
Doctor		Contact	
Location			

REASON FOR VISIT

QUESTIONS/NOTES

DIAGNOSIS/FEEDBACK

PRESCRIPTION/INSTRUCTION

Temperature		Heart rate	
Weight		Blood pressure	

NOTES: _____
_____
_____
_____

Doctor VISIT LOG

Date		Time	
Doctor		Contact	
Location			

REASON FOR VISIT

QUESTIONS/NOTES

DIAGNOSIS/FEEDBACK

PRESCRIPTION/INSTRUCTION

Temperature		Heart rate	
Weight		Blood pressure	

NOTES:_____

Doctor VISIT LOG

Date		Time	
Doctor		Contact	
Location			

REASON FOR VISIT

QUESTIONS/NOTES

DIAGNOSIS/FEEDBACK

PRESCRIPTION/INSTRUCTION

Temperature		Heart rate	
Weight		Blood pressure	

NOTES:------------------------------------

Doctor VISIT LOG

Date		Time	
Doctor		Contact	
Location			

REASON FOR VISIT

QUESTIONS/NOTES

DIAGNOSIS/FEEDBACK

PRESCRIPTION/INSTRUCTION

Temperature		Heart rate	
Weight		Blood pressure	

NOTES:_____

Doctor VISIT LOG

Date		Time	
Doctor		Contact	
Location			

REASON FOR VISIT

QUESTIONS/NOTES

DIAGNOSIS/FEEDBACK

PRESCRIPTION/INSTRUCTION

Temperature		Heart rate	
Weight		Blood pressure	

NOTES:---------------------------------

Doctor VISIT LOG

Date		Time	
Doctor		Contact	
Location			

REASON FOR VISIT

QUESTIONS/NOTES

DIAGNOSIS/FEEDBACK

PRESCRIPTION/INSTRUCTION

Temperature		Heart rate	
Weight		Blood pressure	

NOTES:_____

Doctor VISIT LOG

Date		Time	
Doctor		Contact	
Location			

REASON FOR VISIT

QUESTIONS/NOTES

DIAGNOSIS/FEEDBACK

PRESCRIPTION/INSTRUCTION

Temperature		Heart rate	
Weight		Blood pressure	

NOTES: ---

Doctor VISIT LOG

Date		Time	
Doctor		Contact	
Location			

REASON FOR VISIT

\- -
\- -
\- -
\- -
\- -

QUESTIONS/NOTES

\- -
\- -
\- -
\- -
\- -

DIAGNOSIS/FEEDBACK

\- -
\- -
\- -
\- -
\- -

PRESCRIPTION/INSTRUCTION

\- -
\- -
\- -
\- -
\- -

Temperature		Heart rate	
Weight		Blood pressure	

NOTES: -
\- -
\- -
\- -

Doctor VISIT LOG

Date		Time	
Doctor		Contact	
Location			

REASON FOR VISIT

QUESTIONS/NOTES

DIAGNOSIS/FEEDBACK

PRESCRIPTION/INSTRUCTION

Temperature		Heart rate	
Weight		Blood pressure	

NOTES: _____

Doctor VISIT LOG

Date		Time	
Doctor		Contact	
Location			

REASON FOR VISIT

DIAGNOSIS/FEEDBACK

QUESTIONS/NOTES

PRESCRIPTION/INSTRUCTION

Temperature		Heart rate	
Weight		Blood pressure	

NOTES:-----------------------------------

Doctor VISIT LOG

Date		Time	
Doctor		Contact	
Location			

REASON FOR VISIT

QUESTIONS/NOTES

DIAGNOSIS/FEEDBACK

PRESCRIPTION/INSTRUCTION

Temperature		Heart rate	
Weight		Blood pressure	

NOTES:_____

Doctor VISIT LOG

Date		Time	
Doctor		Contact	
Location			

REASON FOR VISIT

QUESTIONS/NOTES

DIAGNOSIS/FEEDBACK

PRESCRIPTION/INSTRUCTION

Temperature		Heart rate	
Weight		Blood pressure	

NOTES: _____

Doctor VISIT LOG

Date		Time	
Doctor		Contact	
Location			

REASON FOR VISIT

QUESTIONS/NOTES

DIAGNOSIS/FEEDBACK

PRESCRIPTION/INSTRUCTION

Temperature		Heart rate	
Weight		Blood pressure	

NOTES: ------------------------------

Doctor VISIT LOG

Date		Time	
Doctor		Contact	
Location			

REASON FOR VISIT

QUESTIONS/NOTES

DIAGNOSIS/FEEDBACK

PRESCRIPTION/INSTRUCTION

Temperature		Heart rate	
Weight		Blood pressure	

NOTES: _____

Doctor VISIT LOG

Date		Time	
Doctor		Contact	
Location			

REASON FOR VISIT

QUESTIONS/NOTES

DIAGNOSIS/FEEDBACK

PRESCRIPTION/INSTRUCTION

Temperature		Heart rate	
Weight		Blood pressure	

NOTES:--------------------------------

Doctor VISIT LOG

Date		Time	
Doctor		Contact	
Location			

REASON FOR VISIT

QUESTIONS/NOTES

DIAGNOSIS/FEEDBACK

PRESCRIPTION/INSTRUCTION

Temperature		Heart rate	
Weight		Blood pressure	

NOTES:_____

Doctor VISIT LOG

Date		Time	
Doctor		Contact	
Location			

REASON FOR VISIT

QUESTIONS/NOTES

DIAGNOSIS/FEEDBACK

PRESCRIPTION/INSTRUCTION

Temperature		Heart rate	
Weight		Blood pressure	

NOTES: ---------------------------------

Doctor VISIT LOG

Date		Time	
Doctor		Contact	
Location			

REASON FOR VISIT

QUESTIONS/NOTES

DIAGNOSIS/FEEDBACK

PRESCRIPTION/INSTRUCTION

Temperature		Heart rate	
Weight		Blood pressure	

NOTES:-------------------------------------

Doctor VISIT LOG

Date		Time	
Doctor		Contact	
Location			

REASON FOR VISIT

QUESTIONS/NOTES

DIAGNOSIS/FEEDBACK

PRESCRIPTION/INSTRUCTION

Temperature		Heart rate	
Weight		Blood pressure	

NOTES:_____

Doctor VISIT LOG

Date		Time	
Doctor		Contact	
Location			

REASON FOR VISIT

QUESTIONS/NOTES

DIAGNOSIS/FEEDBACK

PRESCRIPTION/INSTRUCTION

Temperature		Heart rate	
Weight		Blood pressure	

NOTES:--------------------------------------

Doctor VISIT LOG

Date		Time	
Doctor		Contact	
Location			

REASON FOR VISIT

QUESTIONS/NOTES

DIAGNOSIS/FEEDBACK

PRESCRIPTION/INSTRUCTION

Temperature		Heart rate	
Weight		Blood pressure	

NOTES: ----------------------------------

Doctor VISIT LOG

Date		Time	
Doctor		Contact	
Location			

REASON FOR VISIT

QUESTIONS/NOTES

DIAGNOSIS/FEEDBACK

PRESCRIPTION/INSTRUCTION

Temperature		Heart rate	
Weight		Blood pressure	

NOTES:------------------------------------

Doctor VISIT LOG

Date		Time	
Doctor		Contact	
Location			

REASON FOR VISIT

QUESTIONS/NOTES

DIAGNOSIS/FEEDBACK

PRESCRIPTION/INSTRUCTION

Temperature		Heart rate	
Weight		Blood pressure	

NOTES: ---------------------------

Doctor VISIT LOG

Date		Time	
Doctor		Contact	
Location			

REASON FOR VISIT

QUESTIONS/NOTES

DIAGNOSIS/FEEDBACK

PRESCRIPTION/INSTRUCTION

Temperature		Heart rate	
Weight		Blood pressure	

NOTES:--

Doctor VISIT LOG

Date		Time	
Doctor		Contact	
Location			

REASON FOR VISIT

QUESTIONS/NOTES

DIAGNOSIS/FEEDBACK

PRESCRIPTION/INSTRUCTION

Temperature		Heart rate	
Weight		Blood pressure	

NOTES: --------------------------------

Doctor VISIT LOG

Date		**Time**	
Doctor		**Contact**	
Location			

REASON FOR VISIT

QUESTIONS/NOTES

DIAGNOSIS/FEEDBACK

PRESCRIPTION/INSTRUCTION

Temperature		**Heart rate**	
Weight		**Blood pressure**	

NOTES: -----------------------------------

$Test$ RESULTS

Date	Test name	Result

$\mathscr{Test}$ RESULTS

Date	Test name	Result

Test RESULTS

Date	Test name	Result

Test RESULTS

Date	Test name	Result

$Test$ RESULTS

Date	Test name	Result

Test RESULTS

Date	Test name	Result

Test RESULTS

Date	Test name	Result

Test RESULTS

Date	Test name	Result

Test RESULTS

Date	Test name	Result

Test RESULTS

Date	Test name	Result

Test RESULTS

Date	Test name	Result

Test RESULTS

Date	Test name	Result

Test RESULTS

Date	Test name	Result

Test RESULTS

Date	Test name	Result

Test RESULTS

Date	Test name	Result

Test RESULTS

Date	Test name	Result

Test RESULTS

Date	Test name	Result

$Test$ RESULTS

Date	Test name	Result

Test RESULTS

Date	Test name	Result

Test RESULTS

Date	Test name	Result

Test RESULTS

Date	Test name	Result

Test RESULTS

Date	Test name	Result

Test RESULTS

Date	Test name	Result

$Test$ RESULTS

Date	Test name	Result

Test RESULTS

Date	Test name	Result

Test RESULTS

Date	Test name	Result

Test RESULTS

Date	Test name	Result

Test RESULTS

Date	Test name	Result

Test RESULTS

Date	Test name	Result

Test RESULTS

Date	Test name	Result

Medication LOG

Medication	Prescribed by	Dose	How often	Time of day	Reason	Date started /Ended

NOTES:

NOTES:

NOTES:

NOTES:

NOTES:

NOTES:

NOTES:

NOTES:

NOTES:

NOTES:

NOTES:

Medication LOG

Medication	Prescribed by	Dose	How often	Time of day	Reason	Date started /Ended

NOTES:

NOTES:

NOTES:

NOTES:

NOTES:

NOTES:

NOTES:

NOTES:

NOTES:

NOTES:

Medication LOG

Medication	Prescribed by	Dose	How often	Time of day	Reason	Date started /Ended

NOTES:

NOTES:

NOTES:

NOTES:

NOTES:

NOTES:

NOTES:

NOTES:

NOTES:

NOTES:

NOTES:

Medication LOG

Medication	Prescribed by	Dose	How often	Time of day	Reason	Date started /Ended

NOTES:

NOTES:

NOTES:

NOTES:

NOTES:

NOTES:

NOTES:

NOTES:

NOTES:

NOTES:

NOTES:

Medication LOG

Medication	Prescribed by	Dose	How often	Time of day	Reason	Date started /Ended

NOTES:

NOTES:

NOTES:

NOTES:

NOTES:

NOTES:

NOTES:

NOTES:

NOTES:

NOTES:

NOTES:

Medication LOG

Medication	Prescribed by	Dose	How often	Time of day	Reason	Date started /Ended

NOTES:

NOTES:

NOTES:

NOTES:

NOTES:

NOTES:

NOTES:

NOTES:

NOTES:

NOTES:

Medication LOG

Medication	Prescribed by	Dose	How often	Time of day	Reason	Date started /Ended

NOTES:

NOTES:

NOTES:

NOTES:

NOTES:

NOTES:

NOTES:

NOTES:

NOTES:

NOTES:

NOTES:

Medication LOG

Medication	Prescribed by	Dose	How often	Time of day	Reason	Date started /Ended

NOTES:

NOTES:

NOTES:

NOTES:

NOTES:

NOTES:

NOTES:

NOTES:

NOTES:

NOTES:

NOTES:

Medication LOG

Medication	Prescribed by	Dose	How often	Time of day	Reason	Date started /Ended

NOTES:

NOTES:

NOTES:

NOTES:

NOTES:

NOTES:

NOTES:

NOTES:

NOTES:

NOTES:

NOTES:

Medication LOG

Medication	Prescribed by	Dose	How often	Time of day	Reason	Date started /Ended

NOTES:

NOTES:

NOTES:

NOTES:

NOTES:

NOTES:

NOTES:

NOTES:

NOTES:

NOTES:

NOTES:

Medication LOG

Medication	Prescribed by	Dose	How often	Time of day	Reason	Date started /Ended

NOTES:

NOTES:

NOTES:

NOTES:

NOTES:

NOTES:

NOTES:

NOTES:

NOTES:

NOTES:

NOTES:

Medication LOG

Medication	Prescribed by	Dose	How often	Time of day	Reason	Date started /Ended

NOTES:

NOTES:

NOTES:

NOTES:

NOTES:

NOTES:

NOTES:

NOTES:

NOTES:

NOTES:

NOTES:

Medication LOG

Medication	Prescribed by	Dose	How often	Time of day	Reason	Date started /Ended

NOTES:

NOTES:

NOTES:

NOTES:

NOTES:

NOTES:

NOTES:

NOTES:

NOTES:

NOTES:

NOTES:

Medication LOG

Medication	Prescribed by	Dose	How often	Time of day	Reason	Date started /Ended

NOTES:

NOTES:

NOTES:

NOTES:

NOTES:

NOTES:

NOTES:

NOTES:

NOTES:

NOTES:

NOTES:

Medication LOG

Medication	Prescribed by	Dose	How often	Time of day	Reason	Date started /Ended

NOTES:

NOTES:

NOTES:

NOTES:

NOTES:

NOTES:

NOTES:

NOTES:

NOTES:

NOTES:

NOTES:

Medication LOG

Medication	Prescribed by	Dose	How often	Time of day	Reason	Date started /Ended

NOTES:

NOTES:

NOTES:

NOTES:

NOTES:

NOTES:

NOTES:

NOTES:

NOTES:

NOTES:

NOTES:

Medication LOG

Medication	Prescribed by	Dose	How often	Time of day	Reason	Date started /Ended

NOTES:

NOTES:

NOTES:

NOTES:

NOTES:

NOTES:

NOTES:

NOTES:

NOTES:

NOTES:

NOTES:

Medication LOG

Medication	Prescribed by	Dose	How often	Time of day	Reason	Date started /Ended

NOTES:

NOTES:

NOTES:

NOTES:

NOTES:

NOTES:

NOTES:

NOTES:

NOTES:

NOTES:

NOTES:

Medication LOG

Medication	Prescribed by	Dose	How often	Time of day	Reason	Date started /Ended

NOTES:

NOTES:

NOTES:

NOTES:

NOTES:

NOTES:

NOTES:

NOTES:

NOTES:

NOTES:

NOTES:

Medication LOG

Medication	Prescribed by	Dose	How often	Time of day	Reason	Date started /Ended

NOTES:

NOTES:

NOTES:

NOTES:

NOTES:

NOTES:

NOTES:

NOTES:

NOTES:

NOTES:

NOTES:

Medication LOG

Medication	Prescribed by	Dose	How often	Time of day	Reason	Date started /Ended

NOTES:

NOTES:

NOTES:

NOTES:

NOTES:

NOTES:

NOTES:

NOTES:

NOTES:

NOTES:

NOTES:

Medication LOG

Medication	Prescribed by	Dose	How often	Time of day	Reason	Date started /Ended

NOTES:

NOTES:

NOTES:

NOTES:

NOTES:

NOTES:

NOTES:

NOTES:

NOTES:

NOTES:

Medication LOG

Medication	Prescribed by	Dose	How often	Time of day	Reason	Date started /Ended

NOTES:

NOTES:

NOTES:

NOTES:

NOTES:

NOTES:

NOTES:

NOTES:

NOTES:

NOTES:

NOTES:

Medication LOG

Medication	Prescribed by	Dose	How often	Time of day	Reason	Date started /Ended

NOTES:

NOTES:

NOTES:

NOTES:

NOTES:

NOTES:

NOTES:

NOTES:

NOTES:

NOTES:

NOTES:

Medication LOG

Medication	Prescribed by	Dose	How often	Time of day	Reason	Date started /Ended

NOTES:

| | | | | | | |

NOTES:

| | | | | | | |

NOTES:

| | | | | | | |

NOTES:

| | | | | | | |

NOTES:

| | | | | | | |

NOTES:

| | | | | | | |

NOTES:

| | | | | | | |

NOTES:

| | | | | | | |

NOTES:

| | | | | | | |

NOTES:

| | | | | | | |

NOTES:

Medication LOG

Medication	Prescribed by	Dose	How often	Time of day	Reason	Date started /Ended

NOTES:

NOTES:

NOTES:

NOTES:

NOTES:

NOTES:

NOTES:

NOTES:

NOTES:

NOTES:

NOTES:

Medication LOG

Medication	Prescribed by	Dose	How often	Time of day	Reason	Date started /Ended

NOTES:

NOTES:

NOTES:

NOTES:

NOTES:

NOTES:

NOTES:

NOTES:

NOTES:

NOTES:

NOTES:

Medication LOG

Medication	Prescribed by	Dose	How often	Time of day	Reason	Date started /Ended

NOTES:

NOTES:

NOTES:

NOTES:

NOTES:

NOTES:

NOTES:

NOTES:

NOTES:

NOTES:

NOTES:

Medication LOG

Medication	Prescribed by	Dose	How often	Time of day	Reason	Date started /Ended

NOTES:

NOTES:

NOTES:

NOTES:

NOTES:

NOTES:

NOTES:

NOTES:

NOTES:

NOTES:

NOTES:

Medication LOG

Medication	Prescribed by	Dose	How often	Time of day	Reason	Date started /Ended

NOTES:

NOTES:

NOTES:

NOTES:

NOTES:

NOTES:

NOTES:

NOTES:

NOTES:

NOTES:

Notes

Notes

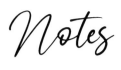

Notes

Notes

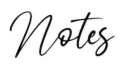

Notes

Notes

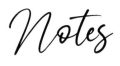

Notes

Notes

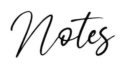

Notes

Notes

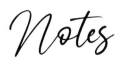

Notes

Notes

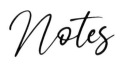

Notes

Notes

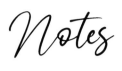

Notes

Notes

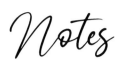

Notes

Notes

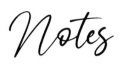

Notes

Notes

Notes

Notes

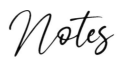

Notes

Notes

Notes

Notes

Notes

Notes

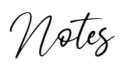

Notes

Notes

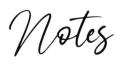

Notes

Notes

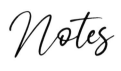

Notes

Notes

Notes

Made in the USA
Coppell, TX
31 October 2022

85531004R10096